Ethical Dilemmas in Nursing

CASE STUDIES AND DISCUSSIONS

M.A. GORRE

Contents

Introduction

Ethical Dilemmas in Nursing

E thical dilemmas are an integral aspect of nursing, influencing not just patient outcomes but also affecting the mental and emotional well-being of healthcare providers. This book, "Ethical Dilemmas in Nursing: Case Studies and Discussions," aims to delve deeply into these complex moral issues, dissecting common dilemmas in various nursing settings and exploring them through case studies and discussions.

Ethics in healthcare is not just about knowing what is right and what is wrong; it's about understanding how to navigate the complex network of patient rights, legal obligations, and moral responsibilities that nurses encounter every day. For example, a patient may refuse life-saving treatment based on religious beliefs. Does the nurse respect the patient's autonomy, or does the nurse intervene to save the life?

Questions like these often have no easy answers and are influenced by a myriad of factors like culture, law, and individual beliefs.

Foundations of Nursing Ethics

To understand the dilemmas that healthcare providers face, it's essential to first understand the foundational ethical theories and principles that guide medical ethics. Deontology, for instance, posits that actions are morally obligatory, forbidden, or permitted irrespective of the outcomes they produce. In contrast, utilitarianism argues that the morality of an action depends on its result; the right action is the one that produces the most good for the most number of people. Different nursing scenarios may be better suited to different ethical theories, and this book aims to provide you with the tools to identify which ethical framework applies to your particular situation.

Legal Framework

While ethical concerns deal with the question of what ought to be done, legal issues deal with what must be done according to the law. Understanding the legal obligations that nurses have towards their patients is critical to ethical nursing practice. This includes understanding the limits of patient confidentiality, the intricacies of informed consent, and the implications of malpractice and negligence. While the law serves as a minimal moral baseline, ethical nursing practice often involves going beyond legal obligations to meet a higher moral standard.

Common Ethical Dilemmas

One of the primary aims of this book is to dissect the ethical issues that nurses commonly face. Issues related to end-of-life care, such as Do-Not-Resuscitate (DNR) orders, often produce ethical dilemmas. Is it ethical to withhold life-extending treatment from a terminally ill patient if the patient or the family desires it? What about resource allocation? In an emergency room setting, who gets treated first when resources are scarce?

Cultural sensitivity is another hotbed of ethical issues. As populations become more diverse, nurses will encounter patients from various cultural backgrounds with beliefs that might differ significantly from their own. How should a nurse approach a patient who refuses a blood transfusion on religious grounds, for example?

Special Populations

While all nurses encounter ethical dilemmas, certain nursing specializations deal with unique sets of ethical questions. Pediatric nursing, for example, often involves decision-making on behalf of minors. In such situations, what ethical guidelines should a nurse follow? Similarly, geriatric nurses face ethical issues related to elder abuse and ageism, while mental health nurses must navigate the complexities of informed consent in a population that may not always be capable of rational decision-making.

Future Challenges and Opportunities

As technology evolves, so do the ethical challenges that healthcare providers face. The rise of telemedicine, artificial intelligence in healthcare, and advanced medical devices like wearable technology, pose questions about data privacy, consent, and the human touch in healthcare.

Objectives of This Book

The primary objective of this book is to provide healthcare providers with a comprehensive understanding of the ethical issues they will encounter in their practice. By studying various case studies and engaging in discussions, nurses can arm themselves with the ethical tools needed to face any challenge that comes their way.

This book is meant to be more than just a theoretical guide. It is a practical handbook for nurses by nurses, providing real-world solutions to ethical problems. From the newly minted RN to the seasoned veteran, every healthcare provider will find something of value in these pages.

CHAPTER ONE

Foundations of Nursing Ethics

Overview of Ethics in Nursing

Definition of Ethics

E thics is a branch of philosophy concerned with distinguishing between what is morally right and wrong, and understanding the principles that guide human behavior. In the healthcare industry, ethics often refers to a set of moral principles and guidelines that govern the conduct of healthcare professionals, particularly in situations where moral dilemmas arise. While ethics is a complex field with various theories and schools of thought, its practical application remains indispensable for providing patient-centered, compassionate, and responsible care.

Importance of Ethics in Nursing

Nursing ethics is a specialized area within the broader field of medical ethics. The practice of nursing is often described as both an art and a science, and ethical considerations can be considered the heart of nursing's artistic dimension. Nurses are frontline healthcare workers who interact intimately with patients, families, and communities. Given the often vulnerable state of patients, ethical considerations are essential to ensure that their physical, emotional, psychological, and spiritual well-being is respected and cared for in an appropriate manner.

Ethical Frameworks and Principles

There are several key ethical frameworks and principles that often come into play in nursing. These include:

1. **Autonomy**: The right of individuals to make decisions about their own healthcare.

2. **Beneficence**: Doing what is in the best interest of the patient.

3. **Non-Maleficence**: Avoiding harm or minimizing harm when benefit is sought.

4. **Justice**: Treating all patients fairly and equally, irrespective of age, gender, ethnicity, or social status.

5. **Confidentiality**: Protecting patient information.

6. **Veracity**: Truth-telling and honesty in all dealings with patients and families.

7. **Fidelity**: Keeping promises and commitments made to patients and families.

Each of these principles carries its own set of implications, challenges, and dilemmas, which are explored in greater detail throughout this book.

Historical Context of Ethics in Nursing

The concept of nursing ethics is not new and can be traced back to the foundational work of nursing pioneers like Florence Nightingale, who emphasized the moral dimensions of nursing practice. Over the years, the field has evolved, responding to societal changes, technological advancements, and new healthcare challenges, such as pandemics, genetic engineering, and end-of-life issues.

The nursing profession has also seen the development of various ethical codes and guidelines. The American Nurses Association's Code of Ethics for Nurses, for example, serves as a foundational document outlining the ethical responsibilities and duties of every practicing nurse in the United States. Similar codes exist worldwide, and while they may differ in specifics, the core ethical principles remain universally acknowledged.

Ethical Decision-Making Models

Making ethical decisions in nursing often involves a structured approach that can include various models like:

1. **The Four Quadrant Approach**: This model helps nurses make decisions by considering medical indications, patient preferences, quality of life, and contextual features.

2. **The Seven-Step Model**: This model involves identifying the problem, considering the ethical principles involved, and evaluating the options before making a decision.

3. **The Nursing Process Model**: This uses the standard nursing process—assessment, diagnosis, planning, implementation, and evaluation—to make ethical decisions.

Summary

Ethics forms an integral part of nursing, influencing not just patient care but also the integrity of the healthcare system at large. Ethical principles guide nurses through the complex landscape of patient care, helping them navigate difficult situations and make decisions that respect both the dignity and the well-being of patients. This foundational understanding of ethics in nursing sets the stage for exploring specific ethical dilemmas and case studies, equipping nurses with the moral compass they need in their daily practice.

CHAPTER TWO

Historical Context of Ethics in Nursing

U nderstanding the history of ethics in nursing provides valuable
insights into the evolution of moral and ethical considerations
that have shaped the profession. One of the most prominent figures
in this context is Florence Nightingale, often considered the moth-
er of modern nursing. Nightingale's work during the Crimean War
revolutionized the idea of nursing from mere caregiving to a disci-
plined profession that emphasized cleanliness, patient care, and moral
responsibility. She introduced ethical norms and standards aimed at
improving patient outcomes and emphasized the nurse's moral duty
to protect and advocate for the patient.

The 20th century saw the emergence of nursing as a distinct acad-
emic discipline, accompanied by the development of nursing theories
and ethical frameworks. Events like World War I, World War II, and
later, the AIDS epidemic and other public health crises, posed new

ethical challenges for nurses, such as issues related to triage, consent, and end-of-life care. These pivotal moments led to a deeper understanding of the need for ethical guidelines in nursing practice.

Internationally recognized bodies like the American Nurses Association (ANA) and the International Council of Nurses (ICN) began to formalize nursing ethics, outlining ethical codes and guidelines to standardize nursing practice across various cultural and national contexts. The ANA's Code of Ethics, first developed in 1950 and revised multiple times since, serves as a seminal text, defining the ethical obligations and duties of nurses in the United States. Similar ethical codes have been adopted globally, emphasizing universally applicable principles like patient autonomy, beneficence, and justice.

Importance in Nursing

Ethics is a cornerstone in nursing for multiple reasons:

1. **Patient Advocacy**: Nurses often act as mediators between the patient and other healthcare professionals. They advocate for the patient's needs, wishes, and rights. A strong ethical foundation is crucial to ensure that patient interests are represented faithfully.

2. **Quality of Care**: Ethical principles like beneficence and non-maleficence directly impact the quality of care delivered. Nurses make numerous decisions daily that have ethical implications, such as resource allocation and treatment options. Adherence to ethical guidelines ensures that patients receive the best possible care.

3. **Professional Integrity**: Nursing is consistently rated as one of the most trusted professions. This trust is built on the

ethical conduct of nurses. Upholding ethical principles in practice safeguards the integrity of the nurse as an individual and the nursing profession as a whole.

4. **Legal Safeguards**: Ethics and law often overlap in healthcare. An understanding of ethical principles helps nurses navigate legal complexities, reducing the risk of malpractice and improving overall patient care.

5. **Cultural Sensitivity**: As healthcare becomes increasingly globalized, nurses are more likely to encounter patients from diverse cultural backgrounds. An ethical framework helps nurses provide culturally sensitive care while upholding universal principles of patient dignity and autonomy.

6. **Moral Distress and Burnout**: Nurses frequently face situations that could lead to moral distress, such as being part of a decision to withdraw care. Ethical guidelines provide a structured approach to decision-making, which can mitigate feelings of moral distress and reduce professional burnout.

7. **Adaptation to Emerging Challenges**: As technology and medical knowledge advance, new ethical dilemmas emerge. A robust ethical foundation allows the nursing profession to adapt to these challenges effectively.

In summary, the historical development of ethics in nursing has shaped the way nurses interact with patients, other healthcare providers, and society at large. The importance of ethics in nursing cannot be overstated; it is fundamental to the provision of compassionate, high-quality care and is crucial for the development and maintenance of trust within the healthcare system. Ethical considerations inform every aspect of nursing, from daily interactions with patients to larger issues like healthcare policy and resource allocation.

CHAPTER THREE

Ethical Theories and Principles in Nursing

Deontology

Deontology is a normative ethical theory that emphasizes the moral importance of rules, duties, and principles, irrespective of the outcomes. In the context of nursing, this approach may often align with the idea of a "duty to care." According to deontological ethics, there are moral rules that must be followed. For example, honesty is a duty: a nurse must not deceive a patient, regardless of whether the truth might be painful.

A significant aspect of deontology in nursing is the principle of autonomy, which upholds the moral and legal right for patients to make their own healthcare decisions. In such cases, the nurse's duty is to provide all necessary information to the patient, enabling them to make an informed choice, even if the nurse disagrees with the decision.

However, deontology can be challenging because it can lead to ethical dilemmas where duties conflict. For example, what should a nurse do if a patient chooses not to take a life-saving treatment due to religious beliefs? Respecting patient autonomy might conflict with the nurse's perceived duty to preserve life.

Utilitarianism

Utilitarianism is an ethical theory that focuses on outcomes, specifically aiming to achieve the greatest good for the greatest number. In nursing, this could mean allocating resources where they will have the most impact. For instance, in a triage situation, care might be provided first to patients who are most likely to survive, thereby benefiting the greater number of people.

One strength of utilitarianism in a nursing context is its applicability to public health ethics, such as vaccination programs, which aim for the greatest overall societal benefit. However, utilitarianism can pose ethical challenges. It might justify actions that are harmful to an individual if they result in a greater overall good, potentially undermining individual patient rights and dignity. For example, is it ethical to prioritize the young over the elderly in resource-scarce situations purely based on the "utility" of remaining life years?

Virtue Ethics

Virtue ethics focus on the moral character of individuals rather than the morality of specific actions. This theory can be particularly relevant to nursing, a profession often characterized by virtues such as compassion, integrity, and wisdom. Virtue ethics asks not what the right action is, but what a good person would do in a particular situation.

In nursing, this could manifest in genuinely caring for patients as individuals, going beyond just performing tasks or duties. A nurse demonstrating virtue ethics would not just administer medication because it's a requirement but would do so in a manner that respects the patient's dignity, possibly taking time to explain the medication's purpose and side effects to the patient. However, one limitation is that virtue ethics may not provide clear guidance in dilemmas where virtues conflict, such as balancing honesty with kindness when delivering difficult news.

Care Ethics

Care ethics emphasizes relationships and caring interaction as a fundamental aspect of moral reasoning. This ethical approach is closely aligned with the nursing profession, given its focus on patient care. Care ethics argues that moral agents have a responsibility to care for one another, emphasizing virtues like empathy, compassion, and responsiveness to need.

In nursing, care ethics may guide a nurse in choosing to spend additional time with a frightened patient, even if it means falling behind on other responsibilities. It could also inform broader nursing practices such as patient advocacy, where the nurse might take steps to ensure a patient's wishes are respected in healthcare decisions. One criticism of care ethics is that it may be too particularistic, focusing intensely on immediate relationships and potentially neglecting broader social justice issues or impartial duties.

In conclusion, each ethical theory offers a different lens through which to examine and resolve moral dilemmas in nursing. Often, nurses may find it beneficial to draw upon multiple theories when faced with complex ethical situations. By understanding the strengths and limitations of each theory, nurses can make well-rounded ethical decisions that respect both individual patient needs and broader societal considerations.

CHAPTER FOUR

Ethical Decision-Making Models in Nursing

Decision-making in nursing often involves complex ethical considerations. To navigate these challenges, several ethical decision-making models have been developed. These frameworks provide structured approaches to evaluate options and outcomes, ultimately aiding nurses in making the best choices for their patients. Below are some commonly used models:

The Four Quadrant Approach

The Four Quadrant Approach is a popular model used primarily in bioethics to address ethical dilemmas in healthcare. This model divides ethical problems into four categories or 'quadrants':

1. **Medical Indications**: What is the diagnosis, and what are the treatment options?

2. **Patient Preferences**: What does the patient want, and have they provided informed consent?

3. **Quality of Life**: What will the patient's life look like after the treatment, and does the treatment align with the patient's values and beliefs?

4. **Contextual Features**: Are there any legal, economic, or social factors that may influence the decision?

Each quadrant must be thoroughly evaluated before making an ethical decision. For instance, if a patient refuses life-saving treatment due to religious beliefs, all four quadrants need to be considered. Is the treatment medically necessary (Medical Indications)? Has the patient fully understood the implications (Patient Preferences)? What is the likely quality of life after treatment (Quality of Life)? Are there legal repercussions for respecting or ignoring the patient's wishes (Contextual Features)?

The Seven-Step Model

This model provides a comprehensive outline for decision-making, broken down into seven steps:

1. **Identify the Problem**: Clearly state the ethical dilemma.

2. **Collect Information**: Gather all necessary information, in-

cluding medical facts and understanding the patient's viewpoint.

3. **Identify Stakeholders**: Understand who is involved and how they might be affected by the decision.

4. **Consider Options and Outcomes**: List all possible options and evaluate the pros and cons of each.

5. **Apply Ethical Principles**: Use ethical theories and principles like autonomy, beneficence, non-maleficence, and justice to evaluate the options.

6. **Make a Decision**: Choose the best course of action based on the evaluation.

7. **Implement and Reflect**: Carry out the decision and reflect on its outcomes, learning for future situations.

The Seven-Step Model is a thorough and systematic approach, making it particularly useful for complex ethical dilemmas where multiple stakeholders are involved, and the stakes are high.

The Nursing Process Model

The Nursing Process Model adapts the standard nursing process—Assessment, Diagnosis, Planning, Implementation, and Evaluation (ADPIE)—to make ethical decisions.

1. **Assessment**: Gather all relevant information, such as medical history, current condition, and patient and family preferences.

2. **Diagnosis**: Identify the ethical issue at hand. This is often

framed as a question, e.g., "Is it ethical to withhold information from a patient at a family's request?"

3. **Planning**: Develop potential courses of action, considering
the ethical principles that apply.

4. **Implementation**: Execute the chosen action.

5. **Evaluation**: Assess the outcomes and reflect on what could
be done differently in similar future situations.

The Nursing Process Model is particularly helpful for nurses as it
integrates seamlessly with their existing workflow and taps into skills
and methodologies they are already familiar with.

In summary, ethical decision-making models serve as invaluable
tools for nurses grappling with ethical dilemmas. Each model offers
a different approach and comes with its own set of advantages and
limitations. Depending on the complexity and nature of the dilemma,
nurses may choose one model over others or even combine elements
from multiple models for a more comprehensive evaluation. Regardless of the chosen model, the ultimate goal remains the same: to make
ethical decisions that best serve the patient's needs while adhering to
the core principles of nursing ethics.

CHAPTER FIVE

Legal Framework and Issues in Nursing

T he legal landscape for nursing is intricate and closely aligned with ethical considerations. Understanding this legal framework is vital for providing safe, effective care while also safeguarding against legal repercussions. The following are some of the most relevant legal issues in nursing:

Legal Issues in Nursing

Legal issues in nursing often intersect with ethical responsibilities, and a solid understanding of the law is essential for nurses. Issues can range from patient confidentiality and informed consent to malpractice and negligence. Legal issues often come into play when ethical considerations are not clearly defined or when multiple ethical principles conflict. Failing to understand or act in accordance with legal obligations can result in disciplinary actions, lawsuits, or even criminal charges. Therefore, it is crucial for nurses to stay updated on laws and regulations pertinent to their practice.

Patient Confidentiality

Patient confidentiality is rooted in the ethical principle of autonomy and is legally protected under laws such as the Health Insurance Portability and Accountability Act (HIPAA) in the United States. Under HIPAA, healthcare providers, including nurses, must take all reasonable steps to ensure that patient information is secure and only disclosed to authorized individuals.

Patient confidentiality extends beyond just medical records to also include personal information disclosed during healthcare consultations. Failure to maintain confidentiality can result in severe legal penalties and damage to the patient-provider relationship. However, there are certain exceptions where nurses are required to break confidentiality, such as in cases of public safety (e.g., reporting child abuse or intent to harm others).

Informed Consent

The principle of informed consent derives from both ethical and legal imperatives emphasizing patient autonomy. Legally, patients have a right to be fully informed about proposed medical procedures, treatments, or interventions. The nurse plays a crucial role in this process by helping explain complex medical terminology in a manner that the patient can understand and by ensuring that the patient's questions are answered.

Failure to obtain informed consent can result in legal repercussions, including charges of assault and battery. It's important to note that consent can be withdrawn at any time and that the patient has the right to be informed about alternative treatments and the potential consequences of declining treatment.

Malpractice and Negligence

Malpractice refers to professional misconduct or unreasonable lack of skill in the execution of professional duties, which can include both commission (doing something wrong) and omission (failing to do something necessary). Negligence is a form of malpractice and refers to a failure to exercise the level of care that a competent nurse would provide under similar circumstances.

To avoid malpractice and negligence, nurses are advised to adhere strictly to nursing protocols and guidelines, maintain clear and thorough documentation, and continue professional development to keep their skills and knowledge up-to-date. Legal claims of malpractice or negligence typically require proof of four key elements: duty, breach of duty, causation, and damages. All these must be established to hold a nurse legally responsible for a patient's harm.

In summary, the legal framework for nursing is a complex structure that overlays ethical considerations in patient care. A deep understanding of relevant laws and regulations, such as those governing patient confidentiality, informed consent, and malpractice, is vital for nursing professionals. These legal principles serve not just as a mechanism for disciplinary action but also as guidelines that promote the best possible patient outcomes and protect the integrity of the healthcare system. It is therefore essential for nurses to engage in continuous education and consultation with legal advisors to navigate this complex landscape effectively.

CHAPTER SIX

Patient Rights and Nursing Responsibilities

N avigating the healthcare system involves a delicate balance between patients' rights and healthcare providers' responsibilities. In nursing, this balance is especially critical given the close, often personal, relationship between nurses and patients. Below are some of the most fundamental patient rights and corresponding nursing responsibilities:

The Right to Privacy

Patient's Right: Patients have a legal and ethical right to privacy, which includes confidentiality of their medical records and the right to have private conversations with healthcare providers. Laws like the Health Insurance Portability and Accountability Act (HIPAA) in the United States enforce these rights.

Nursing Responsibilities: Nurses are responsible for upholding the patient's right to privacy in multiple ways. They must ensure secure handling and storage of medical records and other sensitive information. This extends to verbal communication; discussions about a patient's condition should only occur in private settings and only include those who need the information for the patient's care. Nurses also need to be mindful of privacy during physical examinations and personal care activities, ensuring that curtains are closed and doors are shut to prevent unnecessary exposure.

The Right to Autonomy

Patient's Right: Patients have the right to make their own healthcare decisions, a concept known as autonomy. This includes the right to refuse treatment, choose from among different treatment options, and have a say in end-of-life care.

Nursing Responsibilities: Respecting a patient's autonomy is central to ethical nursing practice. Nurses can promote autonomy through informed consent, ensuring the patient understands their condition and treatment options. They must also respect a patient's choices even if they disagree with them, so long as the patient is of sound mind and the choices don't put others at risk. The nurse's role involves being an advocate for the patient, especially in instances where a patient's autonomy might be compromised, such as with minor patients or those with impaired cognitive function.

The Right to Dignity

Patient's Right: All patients have the right to be treated with dignity and respect, irrespective of their medical condition, age, gender, race, or social status. This includes the right to be free from any form of abuse, discrimination, or degrading treatment.

Nursing Responsibilities: Upholding a patient's dignity is a multifaceted responsibility for nurses. It involves showing respect in all interactions, from how nurses speak to patients to the way they carry out procedures. For example, taking extra care when performing personal hygiene tasks, or offering a patient choices whenever possible, can go a long way in maintaining dignity. The nurse is also often the frontline advocate for the patient in preventing any forms of abuse or discrimination from other healthcare providers or even family members.

In summary, a thorough understanding of patient rights is crucial for nurses to effectively meet their professional and ethical responsibilities. These rights and responsibilities are not just theoretical or legal constructs but form the core of patient-centered care. By actively upholding these principles, nurses contribute significantly to the well-being and overall healthcare experience of their patients. This not only limits legal liability but also enhances the quality and humanity of healthcare delivery.

CHAPTER SEVEN

Common Ethical Dilemmas in Nursing

E thical dilemmas are complex situations where nurses may find it difficult to decide on the morally appropriate course of action. While many dilemmas exist, one area that consistently raises ethical questions is end-of-life care. Below are some common issues and case studies related to this topic.

End-of-Life Care

End-of-life care often presents ethical challenges related to patient autonomy, dignity, and the appropriate use of resources. Key dilemmas may involve whether to continue aggressive treatment, when to focus on palliative care, and how to handle Do Not Resuscitate (DNR) orders.

Nursing Responsibilities:

Nurses involved in end-of-life care must balance the ethical principles of beneficence (doing good), non-maleficence (avoiding harm), autonomy (respecting patient choice), and justice (fair distribution of resources). Emotional intelligence, effective communication, and ethical sensitivity are vital skills for navigating these challenges.

Case Study: Withholding and Withdrawing Treatment

Scenario: An 80-year-old patient with advanced dementia is admitted to the hospital with severe pneumonia. The patient's family is divided on whether to pursue aggressive antibiotic treatment or focus on comfort measures. The patient is unable to voice their wishes due to cognitive decline.

Ethical Dilemma: The dilemma involves deciding whether to withhold potentially life-extending treatment or withdraw from an intervention that may be causing more harm than good. It's a conflict between prolonging life and potentially causing suffering.

Discussion: Nurses would typically consult with the healthcare team and the family to make a collective decision. Ethical principles like autonomy (respecting the patient's past wishes if known), beneficence (improving the patient's quality of life), and non-maleficence (avoiding causing harm) would guide the conversation. Advance directives, if available, can also play a critical role in decision-making.

Discussion: DNR Orders

Do Not Resuscitate (DNR) Orders: These are legal orders that prevent healthcare providers from conducting cardiopulmonary resuscitation (CPR) on a patient in the event their heart stops or they stop breathing.

Ethical Dilemma: DNR orders often create ethical tension, particularly when family members disagree with the patient's wishes or when a patient with a DNR order is otherwise healthy and could potentially recover from an acute episode.

Nursing Responsibilities: Nurses must respect the DNR order as a representation of the patient's autonomy. They are also responsible for ensuring that the entire healthcare team is aware of the order. However, situations may arise where the ethical principles of beneficence and non-maleficence come into conflict with autonomy, such as when a patient's chosen DNR status might result in preventable suffering. Here, nurses often serve as mediators in family and healthcare team discussions, providing information and facilitating ethical decision-making.

In summary, end-of-life scenarios in nursing often present complicated ethical dilemmas. These require a deep understanding of ethical principles, empathy, excellent communication skills, and sometimes, the courage to make difficult decisions. Through interprofessional collaboration and patient-focused care, nurses strive to resolve these dilemmas in a way that respects patient rights and preserves human dignity.

CHAPTER EIGHT

Resource Allocation in Nursing

R esource allocation is a critical ethical issue in nursing, often magnified in emergency settings or during times of scarcity. The overarching ethical question is: How can limited resources like staff, medicines, and equipment be fairly distributed to meet the needs of the maximum number of patients? Below, we delve into this topic with a case study on triage in emergency settings and a discussion on the scarcity of resources.

Case Study: Triage in Emergency Settings

Scenario: A mass-casualty event has overwhelmed a small community hospital. The emergency department has to prioritize the care of incoming patients with varying degrees of injury.

Ethical Dilemma: The nursing staff must quickly decide who gets immediate treatment, who can wait, and who is beyond help. They have to balance the ethical principles of beneficence, non-maleficence, and justice.

Discussion: Triage protocols usually follow an established set of criteria aimed at doing the most good for the most people. Still, nurses may experience moral distress when these protocols mean denying immediate care to some patients. This can be especially true for pediatric patients or individuals the staff knows personally.

Nursing Responsibilities:

Nurses must adhere to the triage protocol as closely as possible while applying professional judgment. They should consult with medical officers and other nurses as needed, always keeping in mind the greater good. Clear and quick communication is vital, as is emotional support for both patients and their families.

Discussion: Scarcity of Resources

Scarcity Scenario 1: A hospital during flu season is running low on antiviral medications.

Scarcity Scenario 2: There's a limited number of ventilators in an ICU experiencing a surge in critically ill patients.

Scarcity Scenario 3: During a labor dispute, nursing staff levels are critically low, affecting patient care.

Scarcity Scenario 4: There is a shortage of available organs for a growing list of transplant patients.

Scarcity Scenario 5: Limited funding in a public hospital restricts access to experimental but promising treatments.

Ethical Dilemma: Each of these scenarios raises questions about how to justly allocate resources. Should the youngest patients get priority? Or those with the best chance of a quality life post-treatment? Is it ethical to consider social contributions or the patient's role in their own health?

Nursing Responsibilities:

Nurses often serve on ethics committees or act as patient advocates in administrative meetings where these decisions are made. They can provide a unique perspective on patient needs, potential outcomes, and ethical considerations. In situations of extreme scarcity, ethical guidelines and frameworks such as the utilitarian approach (most good for the most number), the egalitarian approach (equal access), or the prioritization approach (based on medical need) can guide decision-making.

Resource allocation is fraught with ethical complexities that require a strong moral compass, a deep understanding of ethical principles, and effective communication skills. Nurses play a crucial role in these difficult decisions, always aiming to uphold the dignity, rights, and health of all patients involved.

CHAPTER NINE

Cultural Sensitivity and Ethical Care in Nursing

C ultural sensitivity in nursing goes beyond just acknowledging the existence of different cultures. It involves actively educating oneself about cultural differences, being respectful of these differences in healthcare settings, and integrating cultural understanding into patient care. The ethical dimension of cultural sensitivity comes into play when nurses face dilemmas related to the interaction of healthcare practices and cultural beliefs. This section discusses a case study involving language barriers and a broader discussion on cultural competency.

Case Study: Language Barriers

Scenario: A Spanish-speaking patient is admitted to the hospital for surgery. The medical staff lacks fluent Spanish speakers, and there's a delay in securing a medical interpreter.

Ethical Dilemma: The patient's right to informed consent is compromised due to the language barrier, raising ethical concerns about autonomy and justice.

Discussion: While some medical staff may use informal translation methods such as online apps or asking family members to translate, these are not substitutes for professional medical interpretation. Miscommunication can lead to severe medical errors.

Nursing Responsibilities:

Nurses should advocate for professional interpretation services and culturally appropriate educational materials. They must also document any limitations in communication and strive to minimize misunderstandings through non-verbal cues, if needed. Moreover, the nurses should be proactive in informing administrative personnel about the recurring need for interpreters to serve the linguistic needs of their patient community better.

Discussion: Cultural Competency

Cultural Competency Scenario 1: A Muslim woman prefers to be seen by a female healthcare provider due to religious beliefs.

Cultural Competency Scenario 2: A Native American patient requests the integration of traditional healing practices alongside standard medical treatment.

Cultural Competency Scenario 3: An Asian family insists on using herbal medicines that could interact with prescribed medications.

Cultural Competency Scenario 4: An African American patient is hesitant about participating in a recommended medical trial due to historical abuses like the Tuskegee Syphilis Study.

Cultural Competency Scenario 5: A Jewish patient refuses certain treatments on the Sabbath.

Ethical Dilemma: These scenarios raise ethical issues about patient autonomy, beneficence, and cultural respect. How does a healthcare provider respect cultural beliefs while also providing evidence-based care?

Nursing Responsibilities:

Cultural competency training is crucial for nurses to understand diverse cultural backgrounds and their potential impact on healthcare. This involves not only respecting different cultural practices but also acknowledging systemic disparities that may affect specific cultural groups. Nurses should encourage open dialogues with patients to discuss their cultural needs and preferences and should consult with ethicists, social workers, or cultural liaisons when faced with challenging ethical dilemmas.

Being culturally sensitive and competent is an ethical imperative in nursing. It enhances patient satisfaction, improves outcomes, and upholds the universal principles of patient autonomy, dignity, and justice. With the ongoing diversification of societies around the world, the importance of these skills will only continue to grow.

CHAPTER TEN

Confidentiality and Disclosure in Nursing

I n healthcare settings, the ethical principles of confidentiality and disclosure play pivotal roles in fostering trust between patients and healthcare providers. Confidentiality involves protecting patient information, while disclosure concerns the honest revelation of pertinent information to the patient. This section includes a case study focusing on the disclosure of medical errors and a discussion about HIPAA (Health Insurance Portability and Accountability Act) violations.

Case Study: Disclosing Medical Errors

Scenario: A nurse administers the wrong dosage of medication to a patient, only realizing the mistake after the fact.

Ethical Dilemma: The nurse faces an ethical quandary: Should they disclose the error to the patient and healthcare team, risking legal repercussions and damage to reputation, or should they keep quiet, jeopardizing patient safety and trust?

Discussion: The ethical principles of honesty, beneficence, and non-maleficence come into play. Disclosure promotes transparency and maintains trust, while nondisclosure could lead to harm and violates the patient's right to informed consent.

Nursing Responsibilities:

The nurse must promptly inform the medical team and the patient about the error. Immediate remedial action should be taken to mitigate harm. Following the incident, a root-cause analysis is typically carried out to understand the contributing factors to the mistake and to improve systems to prevent a recurrence. The nurse should fully cooperate in this process, and may also face disciplinary action depending on the severity of the error and institutional policies.

Discussion: HIPAA Violations

HIPAA Violation Scenario 1: A nurse discusses a patient's condition in a public area of the hospital, where they are overheard.

HIPAA Violation Scenario 2: A healthcare worker leaves a computer unattended, exposing patient medical records.

HIPAA Violation Scenario 3: A nurse shares a photo of a unique medical case on social media without the patient's consent.

HIPAA Violation Scenario 4: Medical records are improperly disposed of or not securely stored.

HIPAA Violation Scenario 5: A staff member accesses patient information out of curiosity, not professional need.

Ethical Dilemma: These scenarios challenge the ethical principles of confidentiality and justice. How do healthcare workers balance the need for communication within the team against the patient's right to privacy?

Nursing Responsibilities:

Nurses should receive ongoing training on HIPAA compliance and institutional policies on patient confidentiality. In case of a violation, immediate action should be taken to secure the information and assess whether the breach led to any patient harm. An internal review often follows a HIPAA violation, and the responsible staff may face disciplinary action, up to and including termination and legal consequences.

The topics of confidentiality and disclosure intersect with almost every aspect of nursing, from bedside care to healthcare policy. By adhering to ethical principles and legal standards, nurses can foster an environment of trust and professionalism that benefits both patients and healthcare providers.

CHAPTER ELEVEN

Autonomy vs. Beneficence in Nursing

T wo significant ethical principles in healthcare are autonomy and beneficence. Autonomy is the patient's right to make decisions about their healthcare based on their values and beliefs. Beneficence refers to actions that promote the well-being of others. In the healthcare setting, the balance between these two can be delicate. This section explores a case study on the refusal of treatment and a discussion on medical paternalism to illustrate the tension between autonomy and beneficence.

Case Study: Refusal of Treatment

Scenario: A patient with end-stage renal disease declines to undergo dialysis, fully aware that this decision could be life-threatening.

Ethical Dilemma: The healthcare team, guided by beneficence, believes that dialysis is in the patient's best medical interest. However, the patient, invoking autonomy, is firm in their decision to refuse.

Discussion: The key ethical tension here lies between respecting the patient's autonomy and the healthcare team's desire to do what is medically best for the patient. The principles of autonomy, beneficence, and non-maleficence are all at play.

Nursing Responsibilities:

The nurse should first ensure that the patient is competent and has all the information needed to make an informed decision. They should explore the reasons behind the patient's decision, seeking to understand underlying concerns or beliefs. The nurse should also discuss the case with the healthcare team to see if a compromise, such as a different treatment option, is available. If the patient is still firm in their decision, it should be respected, and comfort measures should be provided as appropriate.

Discussion: Medical Paternalism

Medical Paternalism Scenario 1: A doctor prescribes a treatment without explaining other available options to the patient, assuming it's the best course of action.

Medical Paternalism Scenario 2: A nurse does not provide full disclosure about the potential side effects of a medication, fearing the patient will refuse it.

Medical Paternalism Scenario 3: A healthcare provider decides not to resuscitate a terminally ill patient against the family's wishes, believing it is more humane.

Medical Paternalism Scenario 4: Medical staff discourage a patient from seeking a second opinion, confident that their diagnosis and treatment plan are correct.

Medical Paternalism Scenario 5: A nurse hides information about a patient's prognosis to maintain hope, assuming it's for the patient's psychological benefit.

Ethical Dilemma: These scenarios raise ethical questions about the balance of power in healthcare. Is it ever justifiable for healthcare providers to act in a paternalistic manner, assuming they know what's best for the patient?

Nursing Responsibilities:

Nurses should always aim for a patient-centered approach that respects autonomy while also considering beneficence. Open communication, shared decision-making, and informed consent are critical components of ethical nursing care. If a nurse encounters situations of medical paternalism, they have a responsibility to advocate for the patient's right to autonomy, which may involve bringing the issue to an ethics committee or seeking external advice.

Striking a balance between autonomy and beneficence can be one of the most challenging aspects of healthcare ethics. Both principles are critical for ethical nursing practice, and nurses must be adept at navigating situations where these principles may seem to conflict. Through continuous education, ethical reasoning, and patient advocacy, nurses can help to find a middle ground that respects both patient autonomy and the ethical principle of doing good.

CHAPTER TWELVE

Conscientious Objection in Nursing

C onscientious objection in healthcare involves the refusal by a
healthcare provider to participate in certain medical procedures or treatments based on moral, ethical, or religious beliefs. While
it is important to respect the personal values of healthcare professionals, there is an ongoing debate about the extent to which conscientious
objection can be accommodated without compromising patient care.
This section presents a case study focused on participation in abortive
procedures and discusses the balance between personal and professional ethics.

Case Study: Participation in Abortive Procedures

Scenario: A nurse who has strong religious beliefs against abortion
finds out they are scheduled to assist in an abortion procedure.

Ethical Dilemma: The nurse is torn between the ethical principles of fidelity to their profession, which calls for patient-centered care, and their personal moral commitment against participating in abortions.

Discussion: The ethical tension lies between professional responsibility and personal moral or religious beliefs. The nurse faces a conflict between the duty to provide care and the right to conscientious objection.

Nursing Responsibilities:

In a case like this, the nurse should first review their institutional policies related to conscientious objection, as guidelines can differ. They should promptly inform their supervisor about their moral conflict to explore alternative solutions, such as swapping assignments with another nurse. However, if an alternative is not feasible, especially in emergency situations where a delay could risk the patient's life, the nurse may need to prioritize their professional responsibilities.

Discussion: Balancing Personal and Professional Ethics

Balancing Ethics Scenario 1: A nurse is against administering certain vaccines due to personal beliefs but is assigned to a vaccination clinic.

Balancing Ethics Scenario 2: A healthcare provider does not believe in blood transfusions for religious reasons but is responsible for a patient requiring one.

Balancing Ethics Scenario 3: A nurse is asked to provide end-of-life care that involves administering a high dose of pain medication, which they personally perceive as hastening death.

Balancing Ethics Scenario 4: A nurse feels uncomfortable providing care for a patient who has been convicted of violent crimes.

Balancing Ethics Scenario 5: A healthcare worker is opposed to physician-assisted suicide but works in a jurisdiction where it is legal.

Ethical Dilemma: These scenarios highlight the tension between personal beliefs and professional obligations. Can healthcare providers opt out of certain duties while still fulfilling their professional role?

Nursing Responsibilities:

Nurses must consider their commitment to ethical principles like patient autonomy, beneficence, and justice when weighing their personal beliefs. While many institutions offer avenues for conscientious objection, these are not absolute and often come with stipulations, such as mandatory counseling or educational sessions. Nurses may also consult with an ethics committee for guidance. However, refusal to provide care based on personal beliefs should never jeopardize a patient's immediate well-being or life.

Conscientious objection is a complex and sensitive issue that challenges the ethical landscape of healthcare. Balancing personal convictions with professional responsibilities is not straightforward and often requires nuanced ethical reasoning. By fostering open dialogue, adhering to institutional guidelines, and employing ethical decision-making models, nurses can navigate this intricate ethical terrain.

CHAPTER THIRTEEN

Special Populations: Ethical Issues in Pediatric Nursing

P ediatric nursing brings its own set of ethical complexities due to the involvement of minors who may not be fully capable of making informed decisions. The ethical principles of autonomy, beneficence, non-maleficence, and justice still apply, but they often require modification or special consideration. This section includes a case study on vaccination refusals and a discussion on the complexities of informed consent in minors.

Ethical Issues in Pediatric Nursing

In pediatric care, nurses not only interact with the child patient but often also with their parents or guardians. This triad can create ethical challenges, especially when the interests of the child and the parents diverge. Moreover, children may have limited ability to understand the full implications of medical decisions, complicating the principle of informed consent.

Case Study: Vaccination Refusals

Scenario: The parents of a 2-year-old child refuse vaccinations for their child, citing personal beliefs against vaccines.

Ethical Dilemma: The nurse faces an ethical conflict between respecting the parents' autonomy and ensuring the child's well-being, along with broader public health concerns.

Discussion: The core ethical principles at play here are autonomy (of the parents), beneficence (towards the child), and justice (in the context of public health).

Nursing Responsibilities:

The nurse should provide evidence-based information about the benefits and risks of vaccinations, attempting to dispel myths or misconceptions. If the parents still refuse, the nurse should document this decision thoroughly, as well as any education provided. Depending on jurisdiction and hospital policy, legal avenues like reporting to child protective services may be considered, especially if the child's well-being is severely compromised.

Discussion: Informed Consent in Minors

Informed Consent Scenario 1: A 16-year-old wants to receive a vaccine against the parents' wishes.

Informed Consent Scenario 2: A 14-year-old cancer patient wants to discontinue painful treatment, but the parents disagree.

Informed Consent Scenario 3: A 17-year-old patient seeks contraceptive advice without parental knowledge.

Informed Consent Scenario 4: Parents insist on an invasive procedure for their child that has limited efficacy, against the child's wishes.

Informed Consent Scenario 5: A 15-year-old requires emergency surgery, but both the minor and the parents are unavailable for consent.

Ethical Dilemma: These scenarios highlight the tension between the minor's emerging autonomy and the parents' rights and responsibilities to make healthcare decisions for their children.

Nursing Responsibilities:

Nurses must navigate these delicate situations carefully, respecting the age, maturity, and cognitive level of the minor. Many jurisdictions have "mature minor" doctrines that allow minors to consent to certain medical treatments without parental approval. Nurses should be familiar with these laws and institutional policies. An ethics consultation may be necessary in complex cases where there is significant disagreement between the minor and the parents.

Pediatric nursing adds another layer of complexity to the ethical landscape in healthcare. As advocates for their patients, pediatric nurses must balance the rights and responsibilities of parents, the autonomy and best interests of the child, and the ethical guidelines governing their profession. Through continuous ethical education, collaboration with healthcare teams, and guided ethical reasoning, nurses can make informed decisions in these complex scenarios.

CHAPTER FOURTEEN

Special Populations: Ethical Issues in Geriatric Nursing

G eriatric nursing involves caring for older adults, a population that is often more vulnerable due to a range of factors like cognitive decline, frailty, and social isolation. This vulnerability can give rise to specific ethical dilemmas in geriatric care. This section discusses a case study on elder abuse and explores the topic of ageism in healthcare.

Ethical Issues in Geriatric Nursing

Older adults may have multiple chronic conditions, take various medications, and face social challenges such as isolation or financial constraints. These factors can complicate the application of ethical principles like autonomy, beneficence, and non-maleficence in geriatric nursing.

Case Study: Elder Abuse

Scenario: A nurse notices that an older patient shows signs of physical abuse, such as bruises and cuts, and suspects that the patient is being abused at home by a family member.

Ethical Dilemma: The nurse faces an ethical conflict between the patient's right to privacy and autonomy versus the principle of beneficence, which would call for intervention to protect the patient.

Discussion: The key ethical tension here lies in protecting the patient while respecting their autonomy. There are also legal mandates to consider, such as mandatory reporting laws for suspected abuse.

Nursing Responsibilities:

The nurse should initially assess the situation carefully, ruling out other potential causes for the injuries. If abuse is suspected, the nurse must consult with the healthcare team and consider the legal requirements for reporting elder abuse in their jurisdiction. Ethical responsibilities may include involving social services and legal authorities to ensure the patient's safety, while also considering the patient's wishes and mental capacity to make decisions.

Discussion: Ageism in Healthcare

Ageism Scenario 1: A healthcare provider minimizes an older patient's complaints about pain, attributing it to "normal aging."

Ageism Scenario 2: A medical team decides not to offer a potentially beneficial surgery to an older patient based solely on their age.

Ageism Scenario 3: An older patient is not provided sufficient information about treatment options because it's assumed they wouldn't understand or want to participate in decision-making.

Ageism Scenario 4: A hospital prioritizes younger patients for resource-intensive treatments in a scarcity situation without a clear medical justification.

Ageism Scenario 5: A nurse expresses frustration with having "too many" older patients, considering them more demanding and less rewarding to care for.

Ethical Dilemma: These scenarios demonstrate how ageism can affect healthcare decisions and potentially compromise the ethical principles of justice, beneficence, and autonomy.

Nursing Responsibilities:

Nurses must be vigilant about recognizing and challenging ageist attitudes or practices, both in themselves and others. Ethical nursing care for older adults should be guided by the same principles as care for any other patient, modified only by specific clinical considerations. It may be beneficial to consult with an ethics committee or utilize decision-making frameworks to ensure that age does not become an unjust factor in healthcare decisions.

Geriatric nursing is an area of healthcare that demands a high level of ethical awareness and commitment. Ethical dilemmas in geriatric nursing often revolve around the vulnerability of the population, making it essential for nurses to be advocates for their older patients. By understanding the specific ethical challenges in geriatric care, nurses can better fulfill their roles in providing compassionate, ethical, and effective care.

CHAPTER FIFTEEN

Special Populations: Ethical Issues in Mental Health Nursing

M ental health nursing involves a unique set of ethical challenges due to the vulnerable nature of patients and the stigmatization often associated with mental health conditions. This section delves into a case study centered around involuntary commitment and discusses the broader issues of stigma and discrimination in mental healthcare.

Ethical Issues in Mental Health Nursing

Mental health nurses work with patients who may be at risk of harming themselves or others and who may not have full cognitive capabilities to make informed decisions. The ethical principles of autonomy, beneficence, non-maleficence, and justice often come into tension in this setting.

Case Study: Involuntary Commitment

Scenario: A patient with severe schizophrenia who has been off medication is brought into a mental health facility by the police. The patient is agitated and paranoid, refusing any medical treatment.

Ethical Dilemma: The nurse must navigate between the ethical principles of autonomy (the patient's right to refuse treatment) and beneficence (the need to provide care that is in the patient's best interest).

Discussion: This situation challenges the traditional boundaries of patient autonomy and beneficence. It also has legal implications, as many jurisdictions have statutes allowing for involuntary commitment under certain conditions.

Nursing Responsibilities:

If the patient is considered a danger to themselves or others, involuntary commitment may be legally and ethically justifiable. The nurse should work with the healthcare team to assess the patient's mental state and the potential risks of not administering treatment. Where possible, less restrictive measures should be considered before involuntary commitment. Family members and legal representatives may also be consulted, depending on jurisdictional laws and the patient's mental state.

Discussion: Stigma and Discrimination

Stigma Scenario 1: A nurse feels uncomfortable around a patient diagnosed with a personality disorder and avoids providing comprehensive care.

Stigma Scenario 2: A mental health patient's concerns are dismissed by healthcare staff who attribute their symptoms solely to their mental condition.

Stigma Scenario 3: A healthcare facility places mental health wards in less accessible or poorer conditions than other wards, implicitly signaling that these patients are less deserving of high-quality care.

Stigma Scenario 4: Healthcare staff use derogatory or stigmatizing language when discussing patients with mental health conditions.

Stigma Scenario 5: A nurse doubts the credibility of a patient's report of physical symptoms due to their mental health diagnosis.

Ethical Dilemma: These scenarios highlight how stigma and discrimination can compromise ethical principles like justice, beneficence, and respect for autonomy.

Nursing Responsibilities:

Nurses have an ethical obligation to provide equal and fair treatment to all patients, irrespective of their mental health condition. This involves actively combating stigma and discrimination in healthcare settings, both at individual and institutional levels. Regular training programs that focus on reducing healthcare stigma, along with ethical discussions that encourage empathy and understanding, can go a long way in mitigating these issues.

Ethical dilemmas in mental health nursing often involve complex interplays of ethical principles, legal mandates, and societal attitudes. By engaging in continuous ethical education, adhering to evidence-based practices, and adopting an advocacy role, mental health nurses can strive to deliver care that upholds the dignity and rights of this vulnerable population.

CHAPTER SIXTEEN

Future Challenges and Opportunities

The ever-changing landscape of healthcare is driven by innovations, societal changes, and evolving ethical paradigms. In this section, we will explore the ethical implications of technological advances, focusing on a case study involving telemedicine and discussing the ethical challenges posed by the incorporation of Artificial Intelligence (AI) into nursing practice.

Ethical Implications of Technological Advances

Technological advances offer immense potential for improving patient care but also introduce new ethical concerns. These innovations may challenge traditional ethical frameworks and require a reevaluation of principles like autonomy, beneficence, non-maleficence, and justice.

Case Study: Telemedicine

Scenario: A nurse is providing a consultation via a telemedicine platform. The patient is located in a rural area with limited healthcare facilities. During the consultation, the nurse realizes the patient might require immediate medical attention.

Ethical Dilemma: The nurse is faced with ethical challenges surrounding accessibility, quality of care, and limitations in assessing the patient remotely.

Discussion: In this scenario, the ethical principles of beneficence (doing good for the patient) and non-maleficence (avoiding harm) are in play. The inability to provide immediate physical intervention poses a risk, while the telemedicine platform itself provides crucial access to healthcare services.

Nursing Responsibilities:

In such cases, the nurse should have a protocol for emergency situations that arise during telemedicine consultations. This might involve directing the patient to the nearest emergency service or enabling a rapid transition to higher levels of care. The nurse should also clearly document the consultation, the assessment made, and any referrals or advice given.

Discussion: Ethical Challenges of AI in Nursing

AI Scenario 1: An AI algorithm designed to assist in patient triage inadvertently incorporates biases, leading to unequal care for minority populations.

AI Scenario 2: A machine-learning model recommends a treatment plan that contradicts the nurse's professional judgment.

AI Scenario 3: An AI system used for patient monitoring suffers a malfunction, resulting in harm to the patient.

AI Scenario 4: Nurses become overly reliant on AI for decision-making, leading to diminished human interaction and care.

AI Scenario 5: An AI application handling sensitive patient data is breached, compromising patient confidentiality.

Ethical Dilemma: These scenarios reflect how the integration of AI into healthcare can complicate ethical principles, like justice, autonomy, and beneficence.

Nursing Responsibilities:

Nurses should be actively involved in the design, implementation, and evaluation of AI systems to ensure that they align with ethical principles. They must maintain their skills in critical thinking and ethical reasoning, using AI as a tool rather than a replacement for human judgment. Regular ethical and technical training will be crucial for nurses to keep pace with advancements in AI. It will also be essential to have protocols in place for dealing with malfunctions or discrepancies in AI recommendations.

Technological advancements like telemedicine and AI offer both challenges and opportunities for ethical nursing practice. As advocates for patients and essential members of the healthcare team, nurses have a critical role in shaping how these technologies are ethically integrated into healthcare. By engaging in lifelong learning and ethical deliberation, nurses can help guide the future of ethical healthcare delivery.

CHAPTER SEVENTEEN

The Future of Nursing Ethics

T he ethical landscape in nursing is constantly evolving, influenced by advancements in technology, shifts in social attitudes, and changes in healthcare delivery systems. This section will outline emerging issues in nursing ethics and provide recommendations for future research and education.

Emerging Issues

1. **Data Privacy and Security**: With the digitization of medical records and the rise of telehealth, maintaining data privacy and security is a growing concern.

2. **Genomic Medicine**: The use of genetic information in healthcare introduces questions about consent, confiden-

tiality, and discrimination.

3. **Climate Change and Health Equity**: As climate change impacts public health, ethical questions arise about the role nurses should play in advocacy and how to address health disparities exacerbated by environmental factors.

4. **Global Health**: As healthcare becomes more globalized, nurses increasingly face ethical dilemmas related to cultural sensitivity, resource allocation, and professional conduct across borders.

5. **Interdisciplinary Care**: As healthcare becomes more team-based, ethical questions arise around scope of practice, decision-making authority, and professional responsibility.

Recommendations for Future Research and Education

1. **Curriculum Development**: Ethics education should be a continuous component of both initial nursing education and ongoing professional development. New ethical scenarios tied to technological and societal changes should be incorporated.

2. **Interdisciplinary Collaboration**: Research into nursing ethics should involve experts from multiple disciplines, including philosophy, law, and social sciences, to provide a well-rounded perspective.

3. **Technology Ethics Training**: Given the increasing role of technology in healthcare, specialized training in the ethi-

cal implications of telemedicine, AI, and data management should be included in nursing curricula.

4. **Policy Involvement**: Nurses should be encouraged to participate in policy development at organizational and governmental levels to advocate for ethical practices and regulations.

5. **Ethical Decision-Making Frameworks**: Research should aim to refine and develop new decision-making frameworks tailored to modern ethical dilemmas in nursing.

6. **Global Ethics Standards**: With the increasing globalization of healthcare, research should aim to establish universal ethics standards that respect cultural differences yet uphold basic human rights.

7. **Public Awareness and Advocacy**: Future education efforts should aim not only to train nurses but also to educate the public on ethical issues in healthcare, building a more informed and engaged community.

The future of nursing ethics is bound to be as dynamic as the field itself. Preparing nurses to meet these challenges effectively requires a concerted effort across educational institutions, healthcare organizations, and policy-making bodies. By proactively identifying emerging issues and conducting targeted research, the nursing profession can continue to uphold the highest ethical standards in an ever-changing world.

CHAPTER EIGHTEEN

Final Thoughts

A s healthcare continues to evolve in complexity and scope, the ethical considerations within the field of nursing are more crucial than ever. This text has aimed to provide an exhaustive look into the multiple facets of ethical dilemmas nurses encounter, from foundational theories and decision-making frameworks to specific case studies and emerging challenges.

Nursing is not just about the application of medical knowledge; it's a profession deeply rooted in interpersonal relationships and ethical considerations. Nurses serve as advocates, caregivers, and often as the moral compasses in situations fraught with ethical ambiguity. The role of nurses is expected to expand in the coming years, both in responsibility and in the variety of settings in which they operate. As such, there is a growing need for nurses to be adequately trained, not just technically but also ethically.

Going forward, it will be important for the nursing community to engage in lifelong learning, particularly in ethics. This includes keeping abreast of technological advancements like telemedicine and AI, but also staying grounded in the fundamental ethical principles that have guided the profession for decades. It also involves nurses taking an active role in policy-making, research, and public discourse on ethical issues, to ensure that the nursing perspective is heard and respected.

The intersection of healthcare, ethics, and technology offers both unprecedented challenges and opportunities. By tackling these issues head-on, with a robust ethical framework and a commitment to continuous improvement, the nursing profession can continue to provide compassionate, high-quality care that respects the dignity and autonomy of all individuals.

In closing, the ultimate goal is to combine the cutting-edge advancements in medicine and technology with the timeless ethical principles that form the backbone of nursing. By doing so, nurses can continue to be trusted advocates and caregivers, upholding the dignity and worth of all patients, no matter how complex or fraught the circumstances may be.

CHAPTER NINETEEN

Resources and additional Reading

Books

1. **"Nursing Ethics: Across the Curriculum and Into Practice"** by Janie B. Butts and Karen L. Rich - This book integrates the concept of nursing ethics across a variety of nursing situations.

2. **"Bioethics: A Nursing Perspective"** by Megan-Jane Johnstone - This book provides an in-depth look at bioethics, with a specific focus on nursing practice.

3. **"Ethics and Issues in Contemporary Nursing"** by Margaret A. Burkhardt and Alvita Nathaniel - This text delves

into complex ethical issues in nursing practice, including social justice, and life and death decisions.

4. **"Guide to the Code of Ethics for Nurses: Interpretation and Application"** by Marsha Fowler - This book serves as a guide to understanding and applying the American Nurses Association's Code of Ethics.

5. **"The Ethics of War and Peace: An Introduction"** by Helen Frowe - Though not specifically about nursing, this book delves into the ethics of life-and-death situations that can be applicable to emergency and military nursing.

Journals

1. **Nursing Ethics** - A peer-reviewed journal focusing exclusively on ethical issues in nursing.

2. **Journal of Advanced Nursing** - Includes articles on a wide range of topics including ethics in advanced practice nursing.

3. **Journal of Clinical Ethics** - While not solely focused on nursing, this journal includes articles that often intersect with nursing ethics.

4. **Journal of Medical Ethics** - This journal publishes articles on all aspects of bioethics, including the ethics of medical practice, which is often relevant to nursing.

Articles and Papers

1. **"The Four Principles of Biomedical Ethics: A Foundation for Current Bioethical Debate"** by Tom L. Beauchamp and James F. Childress - This foundational article outlines the four major principles of biomedical ethics.

2. **"Ethical Issues in Nursing: Experiences of Nurses"** by Judith Wuest - A research paper discussing the ethical issues faced by nurses, based on real-life experiences.

3. **"Ethics in Nursing: A Survey of Middle Eastern Nurses"** by Mohamad Alameddine, et al. - This paper focuses on ethical dilemmas faced by nurses in the Middle East, providing a different cultural perspective.

4. **"Ethical and Legal Issues in Emergency Nursing"** by Kathy Torpie - This article specifically focuses on the ethical and legal issues emergency nurses face.

www.ingramcontent.com/pod-product-compliance
Lightning Source LLC
Chambersburg PA
CBHW062246290526
45794CB00006B/2435